# Herniated Disc

## Tests, Symptoms, and Treatments

**Nicholas Gallo, PT, DPT**

# DISCLAIMER

The contents of this book are based on my personal experiences as a Board Certified Physical Therapist and are for informational purposes only. This book does not constitute medical advice; the content of this book is not intended to be a substitute for professional medical advice, diagnosis, or treatment. Always seek the advice of a physician or other qualified health provider with any questions you may have regarding a medical condition. Never disregard professional medical advice or delay in seeking it because of something you have read on this website. Reliance on any information provided by this book is solely at your own risk.

When someone hears they have a herniated disc, they can feel helpless and doomed. The pain that is associated with having a disc herniation can also be extremely frustrating. It can lead to a person altering their lifestyle, resulting in them missing out on events and activities that they love. Currently, the available treatments range from conservative management to surgical intervention. In my time as a board-certified doctor of physical therapy, I have seen incredible outcomes when a patient decides to go for conservative treatment instead of surgery. A study by Gugliotta et al. compared surgical intervention and conservative management for lumbar disc herniations. They determined that, "Compared with conservative therapy, surgical treatment provided faster relief from back pain symptoms in patients with lumbar disc herniation, but did not show a benefit over conservative treatment in midterm and long-term follow-up." These are interesting findings, but people with disc herniations may also be getting pain in their lower extremities, also known as sciatica. Boote et al. have done an interesting study on this topic. They determined that, "surgery generates improved outcomes in the short term, but at 1 year, outcomes are very similar in both physiotherapy and surgical groups." Given the results of these two studies, it is important to know that surgery may help initially; however, for the long term it is not completely necessary. Now, I do not want you to believe that surgery is NEVER the answer. I will go over some instances when a consult with a healthcare practitioner is absolutely necessary because those conditions are out of the scope of physical therapy. What I am saying, however, is that if someone has a lumbar disc herniation, surgery is not their ONLY option.

If I am referred a patient who has the diagnosis of a lumbar disc herniation, I implement a multi-faceted approach to maximize their outcomes. I will go into these treatments in grave detail later, but it is absolutely critical to get a person performing an exercise known as McKenzie extension exercises. These place the spine in the opposite position that leads to a disc herniation and can help provide a lot of relief in the initial phases of their recovery. It is important to progress a person through these exercises in the correct way because they are often performed incorrectly, in which case they are not nearly as effective.

When a patient has been introduced to extension-based treatment, it is absolutely critical to increase their core strength so that they are able to maintain a strong and rigid spine. Having a strong core is essential for recovery. Therefore, I will also go over some great necessary core exercises that I like to implement in the clinic. Finally, I usually approach a patient's recovery by altering their sleeping, lifting, and postural habits. I commonly find that people are placing themselves in compromising positions subconsciously, which leads to increased pain and can hinder the overall recovery process.

The conservative treatment options for a lumbar disc herniation outlined in this publication are proven in the research community and in my own personal clinical experience. I have personally applied these treatment options when working with individuals with this condition as a board-certified doctor of physical therapy. I have personally seen the benefits of these methods, and I want to make them more well known amongst people suffering from this condition.

I also have numerous free educational videos showing a variety of different treatments and diagnoses on my YouTube channel *Physical Therapy 101*. This channel was started to provide free, to-the-point exercises to patients and practitioners. This channel is continuously being updated and provides a slew of information spanning several diagnoses including sciatica, so please subscribe if you are interested. Supplemental information can be found on my website www.physicaltherapy101.net. I am also available for any questions that people have and you can send me an email at nickgallodpt@gmail.com. I cannot promise that I will email back right away; however, I do check that inbox frequently and can help provide some additional answers if questions arise.

# TABLE OF CONTENTS

# SPINE ANATOMY

In order for you to fully understand what is happening during a disc herniation, first I want to discuss the anatomy of the spine. The spinal column is comprised of irregular bones known as vertebrae. Furthermore, the spine is divided into the cervical spine, thoracic spine, lumbar spine, sacrum, and coccyx. The cervical spine is comprised of seven vertebrae and is commonly known as the neck. The thoracic spine is comprised of twelve vertebrae and is commonly known as the upper back. The lumbar spine is comprised of five vertebrae and is commonly known as the lower back. Finally, there is the sacrum and coccyx, commonly referred to as the tailbone.

In the cervical, thoracic, and lumbar spine each vertebra is separated by something known as an intervertebral disc. This name literally refers to the fact that each disc is in between each vertebra. The disc has many functions, and one of them is acting as a shock absorber in the spine. What is significant about the disc is that it is made up of two components: the outside is known as the anulus fibrosus, and the inside is known as the nucleus pulposus. I realize that these are boring anatomical terms, but when I explain this to people, I tell them to imagine a jelly donut. The breaded portion holding everything inside is the anulus fibrosus, and the nucleus pulposus would be the jelly inside.

# WHAT IS A HERNIATED DISC?

Before I explain what a herniated disc is, it is important for you to understand the particular motions of the spine. First off, the act of bending forward is known as spinal flexion. Performing a backward bend is known as spinal extension. These two motions are essential when it comes to evaluating and treating a person who comes in with lower back pain. Some other motions that are important to note are side-bending and rotation. I will go over some specific mechanisms of injury later, but to understand treatment and the cause of a disc herniation, it is important to know how the spine moves.

Now that I have gone over some very basic spine and intervertebral disc anatomy, I want to explain what a disc herniation is. A herniated disc is when a load is placed on the spine that results in the deformation of the anulus fibrosus and causes the gel-like material of the nucleus pulposus to exit the disc structure. Therefore, the medical term for this will be "Herniated Nucleus Pulposus," or HNP for short.

Typically, when people herniate a disc, it can be part of the natural aging process causing disc degeneration or the result of putting a compressive load on the spine. This is also confirmed in a study by Bono et al. They state that "a large biomechanical force placed on a healthy, normal disc may lead to extrusion of disc material in the setting of catastrophic failure of the annular fibers." You may have experienced this when you bend forward to pick something up and start to feel pain in the lower back, which is a very common mechanism of injury. The pain may have occurred immediately or gradually, over time. The mechanism of injury is typically the same: bending forward places the compression on the front of the disc, and it will typically herniate backwards. The disc may also herniate to the side and cause compression on spinal nerves, which leads to something else, commonly known as sciatica pain. In this case, sciatica will be a byproduct of the disc herniation, and it is necessary to treat both. Therefore, in addition to herniated disc treatment, I will include some exercises to help with sciatica.

The combination of bending and lifting will increase your chances of disc herniation. However, when you also include twisting, then you increase your chances even further. In school we learned to "avoid BLTs (bending, lifting, twisting)." When you combine bending, lifting, and twisting, you greatly load the disc, which can further increase your chances of disc herniation. Therefore, if you do not have a disc herniation, then I suggest that you try to avoid these positions to prevent injury. If you already have some type of herniation, avoid doing this as well to prevent the further progression of herniation.

# DEGREES OF DISC HERNIATION

It is very important to know that there are four degrees of a disc herniation. From least to most severe they are: Protrusion, Prolapse, Extrusion, and Sequestered. Disc protrusion occurs when the disc is starting to bulge and the central nucleus pulposus is starting to press on the outer annulus fibrosus. A prolapsed disc is similar to a disc protrusion in that the central material has not left the disc; however, it is still pressing hard against the outer portion of the disc with a lot of force. A protrusion and prolapse are considered incomplete herniations because the central material has not left the disc yet. During a disc extrusion, the central material of the disc has torn through the annular wall; however, a ligament known as the posterior longitudinal ligament has not been damaged. This is significant because once this ligament displays damage, then it is considered the most severe type of disc herniation known as sequestered. Therefore, it is also absolutely necessary to determine the degree of a disc herniation because this will start to dictate a person's treatment and explain their symptoms.

# WHERE AND WHEN IS THE PAIN COMMONLY FELT?

---

Typically, if someone has lower back pain associated with a herniated disc, they can feel pain in a variety of different areas. First and foremost, they will obviously have lower back pain. This will be due to where the disc is herniating to, which most commonly is towards the back of the spine. If the inside material of the disc has fully left the disc, there is a good chance that the nucleus pulposus is pressing on another structure, such as a nerve. This is why it is not uncommon to hear from patients that their lower back AND their leg are hurting.

Typically, if a patient is suffering from a herniated disc-related pathology, they will note several things. First off, they typically have increasing pain in the lower back when they bend forward, which you now know is called flexion. Bending forward increases the pressure of the herniation because it causes the spine to round and place that compressive load on the front of the disc. Another position that increases pressure in this area is when a patient sits for a prolonged period of time. People tend to round their spines, thus increasing the pressure and pain in the affected areas. Since a disc often becomes herniated in this position, staying in the same position after a herniation commonly will reproduce their symptoms.

A lot of the time, a person with a disc herniation will avoid these two positions. It is common to hear "it gets worse when I bend forward," or "I really hate sitting, I have to stand up after a while." This is because these positions commonly increase the pressure on the disc herniation. However, there is one position they may subconsciously find themselves in, and that position is extension. Extension, as we discussed earlier, is known as bending backwards. If a patient has a true disc herniation that is pressing towards the back of the spine, going into spinal extension will give them relief because it causes the disc to go back into place by placing that load on the back of the disc.

If a patient's disc is herniated towards the back and the side, they may become symptomatic in side-bending as well. Typically, you can tell if a person is doing this because they do not walk upright. If you think that you are altering your posture based on your pain, you should look at yourself standing in front of a mirror and make some postural fixes so that you are in an upright posture.

Since there is an association between having a herniated disc and sciatica, it is not uncommon to experience pain in these positions AND to have sciatica nerve pain at the same time. Sciatica is a broad term used to describe radiating pain going down a patient's extremity. This pain may extend to their buttocks or even as far as their ankles. It is common for people to experience increasing lower back pain and sciatica pain as they sit or bend forward. I often hear that after an extended period of time the symptoms become worse because they remain in these positions. Now that you have an understanding of what happens to the spine in these positions, you know why that is the case. The sitting and bending forward positions cause the spine to round and go into flexion, which is a common position to reproduce these symptoms. Some final instances that may reproduce a patient's pain if it is caused via lumbar disc herniation are straining, coughing, and sneezing. These instances place additional pressure on the disc internally and can aggravate a disc-related injury.

# PERIPHERALIZATION VS. CENTRALIZATION

There are two terms that are important to know if you simultaneously have a herniated disc causing lower back pain and radiating pain down a leg. The first term is peripheralization, which essentially means that pain is traveling further from the spine. An example of this would be a person with lower back pain that extends down their thigh and goes into the back of their calf. Peripheralization typically occurs in someone's lower extremity. An increase in this type of pain usually indicates that the condition is worsening. If I am working with a patient in a clinical setting and their leg pain starts to get worse, I immediately stop the exercise because my goal is to never make someone feel worse.

Centralization is just the opposite: it refers to pain that begins to move towards the spine. An example is that the same patient as before begins to experience relief in their calf but still has pain in their thigh and lower back. Then, after further treatment, they experience relief in their thigh and just have pain in their lower back. Finally, they begin to have relief in their lower back and the pain goes away completely. This is indicative of improvement because the nerve root is having pressure relieved from it.

I will go over a basic treatment in the next section. It is very important that you take note of what happens to your symptoms when you do it. If the symptoms begin to peripheralize, you should back off because you don't want to make your condition worse. If your symptoms begin to centralize, however, you know that things are starting to improve. One side note about centralization: sometimes symptoms will centralize, causing the sciatica to improve BUT the lower back pain to worsen. Do not be alarmed by this. It is normal, but you should still progress slowly and gently through the exercises.

# LOWER BACK PAIN EMERGENCIES

---

Before I begin discussing tests and exercises, I want to make sure you know when your symptoms are consistent with a medical emergency. These symptoms should not be taken lightly. As soon as you experience them, you should seek medical attention right away. If you ignore them, you may do harm to yourself that is irreparable. Sometimes serious medical conditions can mimic musculoskeletal pain and it is imperative that these are checked out by the appropriate medical professional.

The first question I always ask people experiencing lower back pain is, "Are you having any bowel or bladder incontinence?" By this I mean whether they are having any issues controlling their bowel and bladder function. This is significant because it is a primary symptom of a condition known as cauda equina syndrome. This syndrome is essentially damage to the bundle of nerves below the spinal cord, also known as the cauda equina. Although it is a rare condition, it does happen and it requires immediate medical attention. Failure to seek help may result in the permanent loss of bowel and bladder control and/or paralysis of the lower limbs. This condition is out of my scope of practice and requires the appropriate medical action immediately!

The next question I ask people is, "Are your symptoms getting significantly worse?" The symptoms that I am most concerned about are whether the lower back pain is significantly increasing. As I have mentioned earlier, it is also possible that a patient's lower back pain radiates down an extremity. It is equally important to know if the pain going down the extremity is also getting worse. Finally, I usually ask people whether they experience losing sensation or strength in the affected lower extremity. If a patient is progressively losing strength and feeling as if the affected limb is getting substantially worse, this is also a medical emergency. It can mean that the nerve involved is substantially damaged and/or the nerves involved are continually getting compressed. Worsening symptoms in the leg may also be the result of cauda equina syndrome. Therefore, this should be brought to the attention of a medical professional right away.

Finally, there are some additional conditions. If you meet them, it is absolutely necessary to get examined by a medical professional first to rule out any of these pathologies. These conditions are known as red flags and are things that I ask about when I evaluate any new patient. Here is a list of some conditions and what they potentially mean:

- Recent major trauma could indicate a fracture.
- Medical history of cancer could indicate a tumor.
- Fever, chills, and/or night sweats could indicate an infection or tumor.
- Night pain could indicate an infection or tumor.
- Unexplained weight loss/loss of appetite could indicate cancer or infection.
- Severe continuous lower back and abdominal pain

could indicate an abdominal aortic aneurysm.

- Compromised immune system could indicate an infection.

There are a few other red flag scenarios where I always encourage people to get evaluated before beginning physical therapy treatment. These have been proven in the research and are essential in giving people the proper care. Therefore, if a patient has any of these symptoms above, I typically suggest that they follow up with their primary care doctor to rule out any serious underlying condition.

# LUMBAR HERNIATED DISC TESTS

Now that you have some background information on lumbar herniated discs and have ruled out any serious underlying pathology, I want to go over some great tests that can be done to determine if what a person is experiencing is caused by a herniated disc. You may have already undergone these tests if you've seen your healthcare provider or you may have seen these somewhere on the internet. These tests are specifically designed to evaluate the neural tissues of the spinal cord. Neural tissues are commonly pressed on when a person experiences a disc herniation; therefore, if these tests reproduce or even worsen a patient's symptoms, it is very likely that they have a lumbar disc herniation.

## The Slump Test

This test is very accurate in determining whether there is some neural involvement in a patient's pain. It is also a very accurate and quick assessment, so it is frequently used in the clinical setting.

1. To begin, the patient will sit up straight in a chair or on the edge of their bed with their head in a neutral position.
2. Next, they allow themselves to slump like they are slouching into bad posture, allowing their shoulders to round while maintaining their head in neutral.

3. If their symptoms are not reproduced, they bend their head forward and allow their chin to touch their chest. Next, they begin to straighten one of their legs and have their toes pointed forward in an ankle motion known as plantarflexion.

4. To further advance this test, as they straighten their leg, they then point their toes back at themselves in an ankle motion known as dorsiflexion.

5. If negative, perform the same steps on the other leg.

This slump test may reproduce your symptoms and you might be asking yourself, "Why

does this happen?" When you are fully slumped forward, you allow your spine to bend forward. This motion you already know as flexion. When you combine this position with straightening out your lower extremity, you tense your neural tissues. If something such as a disc herniation is compressing a nerve tissue or impinging on it, you will experience pain and tightness. Slumping forward also increases that compressive load on the front of the intervertebral disc and can also lead to additional symptoms.

**Straight Leg Raise Test**

Another test that can be used in combination with the slump test is known as the straight leg raise test. This test was the first test to look at neural tissue and is still used today due to its accuracy.

1. To begin, lie down on your back.
2. One leg is raised passively by the healthcare provider until subjective reports of pain or stretching are felt in the leg.
3. To further advance the test, the toes are bent back towards the patient in the ankle dorsiflexion position.
4. This test is repeated on the other side and compared.

The straight leg raise test may reproduce your symptoms due to placing tension on the neural structures. It is not uncommon to experience tightness in the back of your thigh during this test. A positive result is if this amplifies your symptoms. Typically, a person will feel increased lower back pain and/or increased sciatica symptoms in their lower extremity if they are feeling radiating pain.

# HERNIATED DISC EXERCISES

If a patient definitely does have a disc herniation, there are several ways to reduce their symptoms and a lot of times even make the pain disappear completely. This can be done through a series of conservative exercises that are proven both clinically and by research. It is important to make sure that these exercises are completed in the appropriate order and with appropriate form. Therefore, for each exercise that I discuss, I have a supplemental YouTube video demonstrating it so that the technique is performed as correctly as possible.

## McKenzie Extension Exercise for Disc Herniation

If you know you have a disc herniation, there is an important exercise you should perform, known as the McKenzie exercise. This exercise is performed by placing the spine into extension, which in theory allows the disc to move back into place. Any time a patient comes to therapy with a herniated disc, this is the first exercise they must learn to do because it helps reverse the compressive load they have already put on the disc. The idea behind these exercises is that since you are reversing the motion of the spine that causes pain, over time it can cause the disc to take pressure off of the nerve. By going into extension, it is also hypothesized that the force causes the disc to go back into place. I have a supplemental video on my YouTube channel titled "Low Back Herniated Disc Exercises –

McKenzie Exercises for Lumbar Bulging Disc," if you would like a visual aid.

1. To begin, lie prone on your stomach in a straight line with a pillow under your chest. Try to maintain this position for 5-10 minutes. If you experience relief with this position, then progress. If it is already difficult, continue lying in this position.

2. To progress from here, place your elbows under your shoulders and press up onto your elbows. Press up for a count of one and then go back down. Perform 10 repetitions.

3. For the next progression, place your hands under your shoulders now and press up with your hands. Only press up to where you can tolerate and then lower yourself back down. It's important that your hips maintain contact with the surface you are pressing up from. Perform 10 repetitions.

4. The next step is just like the prior one except that now you are pressing up until your arms are completely straight while maintaining contact with your hips. It is common that people shrug their shoulders up towards their ears when performing this. Therefore, it is important to keep your shoulder blades down and relaxed. Perform 10 repetitions.

5. The final position is pressing up until your elbows are completely straight, as before. However, this time you do a big exhale when you are in the press up position.

The primary goal with this exercise is that the pain will begin to centralize and then go away. I'll give you a typical presentation of a patient who has symptoms that are centralizing. If they come in with pain radiating from the lower back, down the back of their thigh, and into their calf, they may initially experience decreased pain in their calf. As they perform more of these exercises, the pain may then disappear from their thigh and only be present in their lower back. Finally, the pain may only be present in their lower back and then disappear completely. This ideal scenario is the goal of this exercise progression.

One thing to note is that this exercise can be varied to focus more on one side of the spine compared to the other. For example, if you have a left-side disc herniation, you can shift your lower half to the left and then perform the progression outlined before. I suggest to people that they play around with what feels the best and what gives them the most relief.

**Standing Back Extension**

There may be times when people cannot lie down on the floor or a surface when they are experiencing their symptoms. If that is the case, they can still do a variation of the McKenzie extension exercise while standing. Although it is not as effective, in my opinion, it can still provide relief because it places the spine in extension.

1. Begin by standing up straight, push your hips forward, and bend backwards like you are trying to look at the ceiling. Perform 10 repetitions.
2. To progress this exercise, place both hands on

your lower back and push your hips forward. Perform 10 repetitions.

3. Finally, if you would like to add some further extension, do a big exhale while pushing your hips forward. Perform 10 repetitions.

When you place both hands on your lower back, you add some overpressure that allows the spine to go into further extension. Adding that exhalation provides additional overpressure. Like before, you want to be cognizant of your symptoms and progress accordingly.

# CORE STRENGTH

One area that is continually harped on is core strength. Your core is extremely important when it comes to maintaining a stable and strong spine. Think of the core as your anatomical belt that supports you throughout movements. You may have seen people wear weightlifting belts in the gym. Their goal is to provide external support. A clinician named Stuart McGill is considered the lower back pain guru. He has done extensive research on core strength. He has determined that by training the core with isometric exercises, you can increase the core's stiffness and rigidity. When someone has a rigid and a stiff spine, it minimizes micromovements at the joints in the spine and prevents pain. Even if their sciatica pain is not directly caused by a disc herniation, it is still essential that they learn this to prevent further injury.

Isometric exercises are exercises that are done in static positions. A good example of an isometric core exercise is the plank. Isometric exercises differ from isotonic exercises in that the length of the muscle is changing with movement. A common example of an isotonic core exercise is the abdominal crunch. Now, I am not saying that you should avoid all isotonic exercises. However, I am saying that from a rehabilitation standpoint it is essential to include isometric core exercises in the recovery process. Therefore, I want to go over some plank variations that have been effective during my treatment of people with lower back pain.

Before I introduce these exercises, I want you to think of the core as a house that has four sides. If one side is weak, the house is not stable and might collapse. This same principle applies to the core, so it is important to be strong on all sides. Therefore, I incorporate core exercises that focus on the front of the core, the sides of the core, and the back of the core.

I also want to go into abdominal bracing briefly. This is when we tighten all of our core muscles simultaneously to protect the spine. Imagine that someone is about to punch you right in the stomach. You will tighten your stomach in anticipation. When I am teaching people these exercises, I always emphasize that they are bracing their core effectively. Initially, it may be difficult, but over time, as they learn this method, they find it becomes easier. When a person performs this abdominal bracing, it allows the protective musculature around the spine to tighten and further prevent movement. That is why it is essential to learn and develop during the rehabilitation process.

## The Bird Dog Exercise

The first exercise I really like to introduce to people to help with their core is known as the bird dog exercise. It is called this because you begin on all fours, hence the "dog," and then you raise your arms and legs, which resembles a "bird." Like the prior exercises, you may have seen other people do these, but not everybody performs them correctly. This is an essential stabilization exercise for the core because it is a very uncommon position that we are not naturally in. When done correctly, it is effectively strengthening the front of a person's core and the back. I have a supplemental video on my YouTube channel titled "Bird Dog Core Exercise Progression," if you would like a visual aid.

1. To begin, go into the all fours position.
2. Perform abdominal bracing and straighten out your right leg as if you are trying to kick somebody behind you. Hold this position for 5-10 seconds and bring your leg back in. Then perform on the other side. Work up to 20 repetitions.
3. Be sure to maintain a straight line with your spine and do not allow your head to sink to the floor.
4. Make sure your shoulders remain relaxed and prevent them from shrugging up to your head.
5. To further advance this exercise, kick out your right leg and extend your left arm simultaneously. Then perform on the other side.
6. This exercise can be advanced even further when an ankle weight is added to both ankles and when you hold a dumbbell in each hand.

When people initially perform this exercise, they have a difficult time not falling over. That is why I always instruct them to straighten their legs first and then advance to the simultaneous leg and arm combination. A common mistake when people perform this exercise is that they raise their arms and legs too high. This creates hyperextension at the spine and can cause pain. I always tell people to imagine their body is a straight line and their arms and legs are an extension of the spine. Keeping everything in line will work the appropriate muscles and should not increase symptoms.

## Plank Exercises

I am a big fan of doing planks for recovery and from an injury prevention standpoint. They help provide stability and can help a patient really strengthen their core musculature. For the following front and side plank explanations, I have a YouTube video titled "Yoga Core Progression for Lower Back Pain - Plank Exercises for Lower Back Pain."

## Front Plank

The front plank is an essential isometric core exercise that strengthens the front of your core. As it is commonly done incorrectly, I always go over how to properly perform a plank when treating a new patient.

1. Begin on the floor on your hands and knees. Lower yourself to the floor onto your forearms with your elbows directly under your shoulders.

2. Contract your glutes in this position and perform abdominal bracing. If this is already a difficult position for you, hold this for up to 30 seconds. Work up to 4 sets.

3. Make sure you keep your spine all in alignment and keep your shoulders relaxed to prevent shrugging your shoulders up to your ears.

4. Be mindful not to allow your hips to sink down to the floor as well.

5. If you need to progress further, instead of having

your knees come in contact with the ground, have your toes in contact with the ground instead.

6. The exercise can also be progressed by raising one foot off the ground to reduce the points of contact. This encourages additional stabilization at the core musculature to prevent the body from rotating.

7. Finally, the front plank can be performed in the push up position. It can be advanced further by raising up a foot off of the ground to decrease points of contact and to challenge the core further.

It is important to make sure the spine stays in perfect alignment, regardless of what variation is being performed. I usually suggest to people that they watch themselves in a mirror or have somebody watch them. Also, maintaining the core and glute contraction throughout the movement is very important to provide a stable core. Neglecting these steps leads to the exercise not being performed properly and the core not being trained effectively. Finally, it's important to not allow the head to fall towards the ground when performing this exercise to prevent straining the neck.

**Side Plank**

The side plank is also a very essential isometric core exercise because it focuses more on your obliques. Just like the front plank, however, it is commonly done incorrectly. When done correctly, it will effectively strengthen the sides of your core.

1. To work your right obliques, begin by lying on the floor on your right side with your right elbow directly under your shoulder.

2. Perform abdominal bracing and make contact with the floor with your right knee and right forearm simultaneously. Contract your right glute in this position. If this is already a difficult position for you, hold this for up to 30 seconds. Work up to 4 sets and then repeat on the left side.

3. Make sure you keep your spine in alignment and that your right shoulder is related to prevent shrugging your shoulders up to your ears.

4. Be mindful not to allow your hips to sink down to the floor as well.

5. If you need to progress further, instead of having your knee come in contact with the ground, have your feet in contact with the ground.

6. The exercise may be progressed even further by raising the upper leg off the ground to reduce points of contact.

7. Finally, the side plank can be performed with your hand and feet making contact with the ground. It can be advanced further by raising the upper leg off the ground to challenge the core further.

Sometimes people do this exercise with their feet stacked on top of each other, but I believe that places unnecessary strain on the ankles. Therefore, if you are doing a right side plank, I typically recommend having both feet resting on the floor with your left foot placed in front of your right. This is repeated vice versa on the other side. I usually let people choose depending on what they are feeling.

# POSTURE CORRECTIONS

Posture is a massive subject, and I have written another publication exclusively on this subject. When dealing with a lumbar disc herniation, however, make no exception: YOUR POSTURE IS SIGNIFICANT. Therefore, I want to go over specific postures and corrections you should make when managing your symptoms. If you want to learn in full detail how to modify your desk and help achieve this throughout the work day, my publication "Posture Pain: Key Strategies to Stay Pain-Free at Your Desk and in Life" is right up your alley.

First and foremost, when you sit for long periods of time, this can cause your spine to become rounded and that, as I mentioned earlier, will place pressure on the front part of the disc. If the disc is already herniated, this continuous pressure of having a rounded spine causes the material of the disc to remain outside where it needs to be. If the disc material is pressing on a structure such as a nerve patients tend to have their nerve pain worsen in this position. Therefore, I encourage people to get up and walk around at least every 50 minutes. If someone gets symptoms before this time, then I encourage them to get up and walk at the onset of the increased symptoms.

When someone is sitting, it is also important that they don't lean to one side or the other. If someone is dealing with a disc herniation that is going back and towards their left side, sometimes they tend to lean away from the herniation. If I see this clinically, I make sure they are sitting evenly on both of their glutes. If they have difficulty visualizing this, I simply place them in front of a mirror so that they can see they are unconsciously shifting their weight. Shifting one's weight to one side or the other is a bad compensatory mechanism that people do naturally, but it can lead to more complications down the line. Therefore, it's important that you are mindful of how someone is sitting. It is also important to note that if someone has a habit of shifting their weight in the seated position, they may also be performing the same postural mistake while standing. Therefore, it is important to make sure these mistakes are not repeated in the standing position as well.

When a patient is in the seated position, it is extremely important to note if they are slouching or not. Typically, a slouching position includes their head forward and their shoulders rounded forward. If you remember earlier, I went over a test called the Slump Test, which places a person in that position to determine if they are having pain due to a disc herniation. If they already have a disc herniation, when they slouch, they are continuously irritating the structures affected in this position. I typically tell people to avoid this posture because over time it can cause bad complications. Just like the progression of the slouch test, if someone is sitting with a common posture where the head is forward and the shoulders are rounded, this is a recipe for their pain to worsen while being seated. It is important to try and keep the head in line with the remainder of the spine, which I cue by telling people to keep their ears in line with their shoulders.

# LIFTING CORRECTLY FROM FLOOR

---

Since lifting something in a suboptimal position can lead to a disc herniation, I want to go into some details on proper lifting techniques. A lot of times people prevent any movement in their ankles and knees and try to lift with their lower back by bending over and rounding their spine. This places a lot of strain and motion on the spinal column and can lead to injury, more specifically a disc herniation. One way to lift something off of the floor properly is by bending the knees instead of the lower back. This causes more motion to be done at the hips, knees, and ankles instead of placing the strain on the lower back. You might have heard, "Lift with your legs," which is essentially the squatting position I am referring to here. Everybody's anatomy is different, so I suggest you play around and determine which squatting position works best for you.

Another way to properly lift something off of the floor is known as the "golfer's lift." This involves keeping one foot planted straight on the floor with your other foot going in the air as you reach down to pick up something. If you do not know what I am referring to, you can get a quick picture of this online. This is another great position that people prefer. According to the research, it also places less stress on the spine. Whether someone chooses this method or the prior method is up to them. I usually give people the option and let them decide which one feels best.

# SLEEPING POSITIONS

One aspect of daily life that I believe is overlooked in the recovery process is how people sleep. If you think about it, we put ourselves in these positions for long periods of time so that we can fall asleep. I realize that we do not maintain these positions the entire time we are asleep and some people move. It is important, however, to be mindful of the correct ways to sleep when dealing with a disc herniation so that you are not doing more harm than good.

**Sleeping on Your Back**

A position that I have found effective for many people who are suffering from a lumbar disc herniation is sleeping on their back with their knees elevated. You may have already discovered this, but try lying on your back with your knees bent and feet flat. Does this position feel better than having your legs flat? If you feel like this position will be beneficial for you, it is easy to try and maintain this position for a while when you try to go to sleep. Usually, what I suggest is that a patient gets into this position and then places pillows underneath their knees so that they can relax and maintain this sleeping position. Having some support under the knees also helps maintain the natural curve of the spine. You can also buy certain items such as bolsters to go under the knees. Many clinics (mine included) have those on offer. Nevertheless, bolsters are not completely necessary to purchase. I have found that using pillows can be just as effective.

Typically, people find this position to relieve their back pain because by having your knees elevated, you place less pressure on the discs and nerve roots. The best way to start with this position is by having your buttocks and feet maintain contact with your sleeping surface. If you want to try and raise the height of your knees, I suggest doing that slowly. Also, if it does not work right away, try it for a few more days and modify accordingly.

## Sleeping on Your Side

If you are a side sleeper, this can be frustrating because your lower back symptoms may increase as the night goes on depending on which side your back pain is located. As we sleep on our side, our hips and spine may get out of alignment and can increase lower back pain. This can pull the spine out of its optimal position and strain the lower back even further. Therefore, I like to suggest to people that they place a pillow between their knees when lying on their side. I want you to try this position. Do things begin to feel more comfortable? Placing a pillow between your knees while lying on your side allows the hips, spine, and pelvis to maintain more of a neutral alignment. A normal pillow can work for this, but I have also had patients tell me that a body pillow was really effective when side sleeping. Therefore, experiment and find out which method is the best for you. In this position you also want to make sure that you are using a pillow to support your head and neck.

Another thing I suggest to people is that they try their

best not to sleep on the side where they experience lower back pain. I have them avoid this because sleeping on the affected side places additional pressure on the already irritated areas that are causing pain. I know that people commonly move in their sleep and shift positions, which can make this difficult. What I like to suggest to people is that they place a pillow or raised surface on the side where they experience their lower back pain. As they roll to that side in their sleep, this raised surface can prevent them from lying completely flat.

**Sleeping on Your Stomach**

Many people like to sleep on their stomachs. I am not a big fan of this position. First off, this tends to flatten the natural curve of the spine, which is not recommended. It also allows the spine to go into a position known as hyperextension, which can place excess strain on the spine. However, as I have mentioned earlier, being in some extension in the lumbar spine can be beneficial for people that do suffer from having a lumbar disc herniation. It is important to note that although it is beneficial, being in that position for an extended period of time may begin to increase pain and should be avoided. Finally, since people typically turn their head to one side or the other, this can lead to neck strains and pains when repeated. Therefore, I usually suggest that people try to sleep on their unaffected side and/or their back as I described before.

If you would still like to sleep on your stomach, then there is a modification that I suggest you make. Since lying on your stomach causes the spine to lose its natural curvature, I suggest placing a pillow underneath your abdomen. This allows a person's spine to maintain more of a natural curvature compared to having nothing beneath it.

One other modification that can be made to prevent the turning of the head during stomach sleeping is placing a rolled up towel underneath the forehead. This should be done in addition to the pillow underneath the stomach to provide breathing room for the person. Although this may seem abnormal, this position really helps maintain alignment when sleeping on the stomach.

Finally, if you have a softer mattress, this tends to allow the lower back to move into more of a hyperextension compared to a firmer mattress. Therefore, I suggest that people look at a firmer mattress, which I will discuss in more detail next.

# SLEEPING SURFACE

This is a highly variable topic among people that have lower back pain associated with a herniated disc. I have heard everything from sleeping on the floor, sleeping in a recliner, to sleeping on all types of different mattresses. One is not necessarily better than the other because every person is unique. What I can suggest is that you try out several and see how you feel in the morning. When people initially come to me, I have them rate their pain on a scale of 1 to 10, with 1 being the lowest and 10 being the highest. I want you to do the same with regards to your sleeping surface. If you feel improvement, take note and try to modify further so that you are completely comfortable and can sleep well during the entire night.

I also commonly get questions regarding mattress types. Just like sleeping positions and sleeping surfaces, this is very subjective. I have people that swear by certain mattress types and others that I cannot give a specific recommendation on this. What I can suggest is that there are so many out there that if you are looking to purchase a new one, you should go try out as many as you can and make a decision. One option that can provide many possibilities are the mattresses of which you can adjust the firmness. I do not personally have a lot of experience with these and I have read that they can be very expensive, but varying the firmness can be very effective. This makes sense in that you can give yourself a custom setting that you continually adjust until it is perfect for your body.

# SCIATICA TREATMENT

As I have mentioned earlier, sciatica can become a symptom of a lumbar disc herniation. If this is the case, you feel lower back pain and pain that is consistent with sciatica. I will not go into grave detail regarding sciatica because I have another publication that discusses the specifics of sciatica. I will however list some great sciatica stretches and strengthening exercises that I have found to be effective when treating this condition. You can find all the ones I mention in a video on my YouTube channel titled "Exercises to Help with Sciatica During Pregnancy." This video was recorded for a colleague's wife because she was experiencing sciatica pain during pregnancy, but they are effective exercises that can work for anybody in this condition. (Note: the video also features other exercises and variations that you are free to try. I will only talk about the ones that have worked best in my experience.)

## Gluteal Stretches

One thing that is important when dealing with sciatica nerve pain is that you keep the tissues surrounding the sciatic nerve stretched and limber. It is important to remember that, when doing these stretches, you may start to feel some sciatica nerve pain. This is normal; however, you do not want to overstretch these tissues because overstretching can lead to more intense flare-ups of the nerve. Therefore, when you are stretching, you should stretch to the point RIGHT BEFORE you start to experience pain. Always let your symptoms be the judge of how far to stretch, as you do not want them to make you feel worse.

## Single Knee to Chest Stretch

This stretch is performed just like the name suggests: you literally pull one knee to your chest. However, there are a few modifications that are important to try and prevent this from causing additional pain.

1. Lie on your back with both of your knees bent and feet resting flat on the floor.
2. In order to stretch the right side, cup your hands behind your right thigh and pull your knee gently to your chest.
3. If this is too intense or you have trouble grabbing behind your thigh, you can grab towards your leg where the shin meets your knee.
4. If this is also too difficult, you can place a strap behind your right thigh and pull the leg into position using the strap.
5. Perform 3-4 repetitions and hold for 20-30 seconds.
6. Once you have stretched your right side, perform this exercise on the left.

## Piriformis Stretch

The piriformis is a muscle located on the pelvis that can play a major role in sciatica nerve pain. What's significant is its location with regards to the sciatic nerve. If the piriformis muscle is tight or goes into spasm, it can compress on the sciatic nerve and cause pain. In order to prevent this, it is important to keep the muscle stretched.

**Seated Piriformis Stretch**

1. Begin by sitting in a sturdy chair.
2. To begin stretching the right side, cross your legs so that your right ankle is resting on the top of your left thigh.
3. To further intensify this stretch, try to push down your right knee so that your knee is parallel with the floor, creating a "Figure 4" position.
4. You can advance this stretch even further by maintaining an upright seated position and by leaning forward.
5. You should feel this stretch in your right hip and glute area.
6. Perform 3-4 repetitions and hold for 20-30 seconds.
7. Once you have stretched your right side, perform it on the left.

I like showing people this stretch in the seated position because they can do it everywhere, especially if they are at work and begin to feel pain.

**Supine Piriformis Stretch**

The piriformis stretch can also be performed when lying down supine, and I encourage you to do this version as well. If lying on the floor is uncomfortable, you can perform it in bed.

1. Begin by lying on your back with both of your knees bent and feet flat on the floor.

2. To stretch your right side, cross your legs so that your right ankle is resting on the top of your left thigh, creating that same "Figure 4" position as before.

3. Using your hands, pull your left thigh towards your chest while your right ankle remains on your left thigh.

4. If this is difficult, you can wrap a strap around your left thigh and pull on the strap with your hands.

5. Pull until you feel a stretch in your right hip and glute area.

6. Perform 3-4 repetitions and hold for 20-30 seconds.

7. Once you have stretched your right side, perform it on the left.

In the supine position, this exercise can be performed quickly in bed. I like to add it as the next progression to the seated exercise because this one can be more intense than that one. Therefore, I suggest trying the seated version first and then this one after the seated version becomes too easy.

# GLUTEAL STRENGTH

---

I have gone over stretching the tissues surrounding the sciatic nerve. However, it is very important that the muscles surrounding it are strong too. There are three different types of gluteal muscles: gluteus maximus, gluteus minimus, and gluteus medius. They all play a major role in the stabilization of the pelvis and hip movements. If they are weak, a patient will begin to compensate and have exacerbation of their pain. Therefore, I will go over a few of the gluteal strengthening exercises that I commonly prescribe to patients.

## Supine Bridges

The bridge exercise is very beneficial when rehabilitating sciatica. It is an easy-to-do, low-impact exercise that really isolates the gluteal muscles. It can also be done without any equipment and be advanced fairly easily.

1. Start by lying on your back with your hands by your side and feet flat on the floor.
2. Tighten your core and buttock muscles.
3. Raise your bottom up until you create a straight line going from your shoulders to your knees.
4. Slowly allow your bottom to come back down.
5. Work up to 3 sets of 10 repetitions.

This exercise is simultaneously working your core,

lower back, and gluteal muscles. Initially, this exercise may seem tough, but over time you will notice that it becomes easier. When this happens, it is important to advance the exercise to make it more difficult. One great way to do this is, instead of performing the bridge exercise with two feet, performing it with one foot. This is much more difficult than it sounds, and it is a great way to advance the exercise. If it is initially too hard, try doing the bridge exercise with both feet and then raising one while maintaining your hips at the same height. If you notice that your hips begin to fall back to the surface, then you have identified that you need to work on additional gluteal weakness.

**The Side-Lying Clamshell**

This exercise is most often prescribed because it allows strengthening of the gluteal muscles in a different plane of movement. It is also very low-impact; however, it will isolate the gluteus medius muscle effectively, which is important in the rehabilitation process for sciatica.

1. Start by lying on your side with the hip that you want to strengthen facing up.
2. Make sure your legs are stacked on top of each other and your knees are bent.
3. During the exercise, it's important to make sure your core is tight and engaged.
4. While keeping your feet touching, raise your top knee as high as you can without allowing your hips to rotate. If this is difficult for you, lie on your side with your back touching a wall to prevent movement.

5. Pause at the top and return to the starting position under control. Work up to 30 repetitions.
6. Repeat on the other side.
7. When it becomes too easy, add a resistance band around your thighs to make it harder.

I love this exercise because the gluteus medius muscle is so important for the rehabilitation of a patient with sciatica and lower back pain. Most commonly, as I mentioned above, people rotate their hips and the exercise will be ineffective. That is why it is of the utmost importance to make sure that you do not make that mistake.

## Sciatic Nerve Mobilization

Now that the surrounding tissues are stretched, it's important to perform some dynamic exercises that allow the sciatic nerve to be mobilized. Jeong et al. determined that, "Application of mobilization techniques for the sciatic nerves may promote healing of the soft tissues by stimulating the functions of the nervous system to improve nervous system adaptability and decrease sensitivity, helping to alleviate the symptoms." The group that experienced the most relief in this study performed these mobilization techniques in addition to other therapy exercises for lumbar stabilization. Therefore, I like to include these in my treatment plan along with some other treatments I will go over shortly.

It is important for you to realize that you can absolutely overstretch and cause additional pain with these exercises. That is why I always tell people to perform them right before they begin to feel pain and discomfort. The tissues being stretched and mobilized during these exercises are very sensitive, and flaring them up more is not the goal here. You also do not want to do more than 10 repetitions per day due to the sensitive nature of these exercises. I have recorded them in a video on my YouTube channel titled "Sciatic Nerve Glides – Sciatic Nerve Entrapment Sciatica Pain Relief."

**Seated Sciatic Nerve Glides**

A sciatic nerve glide is a technique used to help mobilize the sciatic nerve. What makes nerve glides different is that the nerve is mobilized via dynamic stretching. The first one I want to go over is the seated sciatic nerve glide because it can be done pretty much anywhere and at any time. This nerve glide may seem familiar to you because it is exactly the same position as the slump test I reviewed earlier. If you feel sciatica on one side of your body, perform this exercise on that side. However, I encourage people to do it on both sides because it helps keep them symmetrical.

1. To begin, sit up straight on a chair or on the edge of your bed with your head in a neutral position.

2. Next, straighten your leg with your toes pointed forward. If you are already feeling a reproduction of your symptoms, straighten your leg right before you begin to feel your symptoms and then allow your leg to bend back to the starting position.

3. To increase the intensity, straighten your leg and

bend your toes back towards you.

4.  If you would like to intensify this mobilization even further, allow your shoulders and head to slouch forward and repeat the previous step.

5.  It is important to remember to not overstretch during this exercise.

## Supine Sciatic Nerve Glides

The same mobilization technique can be done while lying supine. Like before, if you are not comfortable doing this on the floor, you can do it while lying in bed.

1.  To begin, lie on your back with both knees bent.

2.  Pull the affected thigh towards you until it is perpendicular to the ceiling.

3.  In this position, allow your leg to straighten, with the toes pointing towards the ceiling. If you are already feeling a reproduction of your symptoms, straighten your leg right before you begin to feel your symptoms and then allow your leg to bend again to the starting position.

4.  To increase the intensity, straighten your leg and bend your toes back towards you.

5.  If you would like to intensify this mobilization even further, lift your head to your chest and repeat the prior steps.

6.  Once again, DO NOT overstretch.

# HEAT OR ICE?

When I am treating people for a lumbar disc herniation, I commonly get asked which is better: heat or ice? Everybody is so different that a "one-size-fits-all" approach does not always work, but I will explain what I was taught in school. Typically, if you want to reduce inflammation, ice should be used. This is best applied during the acute phase of an injury, which spans 3-7 days. After this inflammatory period, it is suggested that you start to use heat to enhance blood flow to the area and to promote healing. Heat and ice should be applied for approximately 15-20 minutes and can be performed multiple times per day as needed. These are good guidelines for the most part, but I would like to include some specifics that I have learned in my clinical experience.

When a patient initially injures their lower back, I would encourage them to use ice, and this is no different when a person has an acute disc herniation. It is important to apply ice to try and calm the tissues down and to reduce that inflammatory response. If someone is having sciatica symptoms and the pain is traveling away from the spine down the leg, for example, I also encourage the use of ice to help calm down the nerve. Typically, heat tends to feel good, but over time it can lead to more irritation. There are times, however, when I will use heat first.

If a patient is dealing with a chronic condition, for

example, having lower back pain for months, I have seen success providing them with heat first. Using heat before a patient starts stretching and/or doing activities can loosen up tight tissues and allow them to stretch more easily. Heat also tends to allow tight muscles around the sciatic nerve to relax, thus decreasing compression on it. I usually do this if someone has been dealing with this injury for a long time and it is considered a chronic injury. After a person has completed their treatment session, if they have increased nerve symptoms and they have increased sciatica pain, I provide them with ice to try and calm the sciatic nerve back down. This tends to decrease inflammation around the nerve, and it may numb the pain. It is not the same for every person, however, so I suggest that you start with this method and then play around with what works best for you.

There are also a few important things to avoid if you are using these methods for pain

relief. First off, always use a towel or some sort of barrier between the ice or heat and your skin. I have seen people burn themselves and nearly get frostbite by avoiding this rule, which is completely avoidable! Also, try not to fall asleep when using these methods because ideally, they should be used for 15-20 minutes at a time. If you fall asleep, you may also damage your skin. One thing I really want to suggest is that you set an alarm to time yourself just in case you do fall asleep. Also, DO NOT stretch directly after applying ice therapy because this temporarily decreases the pliability of muscles.

# CLOSING THOUGHTS

———

I hope that by reading this guide and performing the exercises you no longer feel helpless and lost in this entire process of having a lumbar disc herniation. If you are suffering from lower back pain, it can be easy to feel discouraged and doomed. I have seen people alter their entire lives around this condition because they feel absolutely lost. This can be a horrible condition that I have firsthand seen sideline people for a long period of time. If you have the right guidance and are incorporating up-to-date treatments, then relief can absolutely be experienced without surgery. In several cases that I have treated over the years, I have seen people become pain-free and get back to their daily activities without having to think about pain anymore.

One of my passions as a physical therapist is to put treatment in the person's hands and show them what to do to accomplish this. I really want to make sure that people can become independent when dealing with their ailments. People can accomplish this goal if they truly put in the work and listen to those that have the experience and knowledge. I hope that you find the information in this guide helpful because my goal is to help those suffering from a lumbar disc herniation. I want to help people get back to living their lives pain-free because that is what I love doing day in and day out.

One thing I will add is that if you use these treatments

and start to feel better, just remember to keep up with the exercises and stretches to prevent the pain from coming back. A common theme in the physical therapy world is that once people get relief, they start to slack off with their exercises. Although not all the time, sometimes people start back at square one if they re-injure themselves. I hope that you have enjoyed what I had to say and I want to thank you for reading my suggestions on this subject.

# REFERENCES

Bono CM, Wisneski R, Garfin SR. Lumbar disc herniations. In: Herkowitz HN, Garfin SR, Eismont FJ, Bell GR, Balderston RA, editors. The Spine. 5th ed. Philadelphia, PA: Saunders; 2006.

Boote J, Newsome R, Reddington M, Cole A, Dimairo M. Physiotherapy for Patients with Sciatica Awaiting Lumbar Micro-discectomy Surgery: A Nested, Qualitative Study of Patients' Views and Experiences. Physiother Res Int. 2016;22(3):e1665.

Brinjikji W, Luetmer PH, Comstock B, et al. Systematic Literature Review of Imaging Features of Spinal Degeneration in Asymptomatic Populations. *AJNR Am J Neuroradiol.* 2014;36(4):811-6.

Dutton, M. (2012). *Orthopaedic Examination, Evaluation, and Intervention.* New York: McGraw Hill Medical.

Gugliotta M, da Costa BR, Dabis E, *et al* Surgical versus conservative treatment for lumbar disc herniation: a prospective cohort study*BMJ Open* 2016;6:e012938. doi: 10.1136/bmjopen-2016-012938

Jeong UC, Kim CY, Park YH, Hwang-Bo G, Nam CW. The Effects of Self-Mobilization Techniques for the Sciatic Nerves on Physical Functions and Health of Low Back Pain Patients With Lower Limb Radiating Pain. *J Phys Ther Sci.* 2016;28(1):46-50.

Kauppila LI, McAlindon T, Evans S, Wilson PW, Kiel D, Felson DT. Disc Degeneration/Back Pain and Calcification of the Abdominal Aorta. A 25-Year Follow-Up Study in Framingham. Spine (Phila Pa 1976). 1997;22:1642-1647, discussion 1648-9. 47.

Koes BW, van Tulder MW, Peul WC. Diagnosis and Treatment of Sciatica. *BMJ.* 2007;334(7607):1313-7.

Xiang A, Xu M, Liang Y, Wei J, Liu S. Immediate Relief of Herniated Lumbar Disc-Related Sciatica by Ankle Acupuncture: A Study Protocol for a Randomized Controlled Clinical Trial. *Medicine (Baltimore).* 2017;96(51):e9191.

Wang D, Nasto LA, Roughley P, et al. Spine Degeneration in a Murine Model of Chronic Human Tobacco Smokers. Osteoarthritis Cartilage. 2012;20(8):896-905. 50.

# ABOUT THE AUTHOR

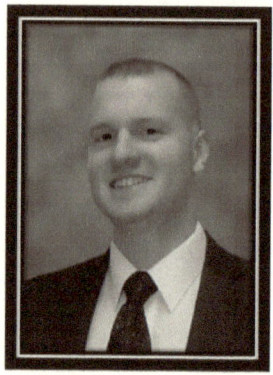

Nicholas Gallo is a board-certified doctor of physical therapy. He has helped countless patients in his career and continues to practice physical therapy on a full-time basis. He is also a cofounder of *Physical Therapy 101*.

# ADDITIONAL RESOURCES

---

For more information, visit my website at www.physicaltherapy101.net. Here we have resources on various pathologies. This website is continuously updated to provide up to date treatment and is a great resource for practitioners, patients, and prospective Physical Therapists.

Subscribe to my YouTube channel https://www.youtube.com/c/PhysicalTherapy101.

Here we produce free treatment videos for patients and healthcare providers. This is also a great visual aid for treatments described above.

I have other publications that you may also find interesting:

Posture Pain: Key Strategies to Stay Pain Free at Your Desk and in Life – I discuss the optimal computer station setup to maintaining ideal posture, exercises to perform to reduce pain, and ways to implement these strategies in other scenarios.

Getting Into Physical Therapy School: 10 Essential Things You Must Do - If you are interested in a career in Physical Therapy this is the guide for you. I go in depth on key strategies on how to get accepted into a Physical Therapy program. These strategies will strengthen your application and separate you from the competition.

Proper Bench Press Form: The Beginner's Guide to Warm-Up, Technique, and Injury Prevention - If you are a beginner to bench pressing or you are experienced but want to incorporate some injury prevention this is for you. You will learn how to warm up properly, ideal technique, and proven exercises to help with injury prevention.

Sciatica Nerve Pain: Symptoms, Tests, and Treatments for Lumbar Radiculopathy – In this publication I discuss Sciatica pain by giving a detailed explanation of the anatomical components involved and the causes. I then show how to properly diagnose the condition and treat it using conservative treatments proven in the research community and in the clinical setting.

Tennis Elbow Pain: Symptoms, Tests, and Treatments for Lateral Epicondylitis – In this publication I discuss Tennis Elbow by going into anatomical detail for the structures involved for this condition. I then lay out a systematic approach to recovery. Once again, everything is supported via the research and my clinical experience.

P.S. If you have enjoyed this book and found it resourceful, please leave a helpful review on Amazon.